Heart Palpitations Relief

A Beginner's Quick Start Guide to Managing Heart Palpitations Naturally Through Diet, with Sample Recipes

mf

Disclaimer

By reading this disclaimer, you are accepting the terms of the disclaimer in full. If you disagree with this disclaimer, please do not read the guide.

All of the content within this guide is provided for informational and educational purposes only, and should not be accepted as independent medical or other professional advice. The author is not a doctor, physician, nurse, mental health provider, or registered nutritionist/dietician. Therefore, using and reading this guide does not establish any form of a physician-patient relationship.

Always consult with a physician or another qualified health provider with any issues or questions you might have regarding any sort of medical condition. Do not ever disregard any qualified professional medical advice or delay seeking that advice because of anything you have read in this guide. The information in this guide is not intended to be any sort of medical advice and should not be used in lieu of any medical advice by a licensed and qualified medical professional.

The information in this guide has been compiled from a variety of known sources. However, the author cannot attest to or guarantee the accuracy of each source and thus should not be held liable for any errors or omissions.

Table of Contents

Introduction   6

The Basics of Heart Palpitations   8

    Causes   9

    Risk Factors   10

    Symptoms of Heart Palpitations   10

Diagnosis and Treatment   11

Managing Your Heart Palpitations—the Right Way   13

Managing Heart Palpitations Through Diet   18

    Foods to Avoid   20

Sample Recipes   24

    Salmon and Asparagus   25

    Tahini Salmon   26

    Seafood Stew   28

    Lemon-Baked Salmon   29

    Salmon with Avocados and Brussels Sprout   31

    Asparagus with Garlic and Onions   34

    Broccoli-Kale with Avocado Toppings Rice Bowl   35

    Stir Fry Broccoli, Onions, and Carrots   36

    Apple and Onion Mix   37

    Hearty Chicken Salad with Pasta   38

    Chicken Breast Delight   39

    Roast Broccoli and Salmon   40

    Oat and Blueberry Pancakes with Yogurt   42

    Apple-and-Honeydew Smoothie   43

    Anti-Diabetic Smoothie   44

    Vegetable Pasta in Avocado Sauce   45

Conclusion   47

References and Helpful Links   48

Introduction

Heart palpitations are a common health complaint in which the heart beats irregularly or rapidly.

There are many possible causes for heart palpitations, which include anxiety, caffeine, tobacco use, alcohol consumption, a sedentary lifestyle, stress, and electrolyte imbalances.

Heart palpitations are also associated with a poor diet because the foods we eat affect how our hearts work. This can lead to many other problems, but the good news is that it's possible to eat heart-healthy foods and reduce your risk for heart palpitations.

This beginner's quick start guide provides information on how to do just that with a heart-healthy diet, as well as lifestyle changes and other home remedies.

In this guide, you will discover:

- The basics about heart palpitations
- Symptoms and risk factors of this sensation

- Diagnosing and treating palpitations
- Managing the palpitations
- Foods to eat and avoid for a heart-healthy diet

The Basics of Heart Palpitations

A heart palpitation, or "heart flutter" as it's also called, is a feeling that your heart is racing out of control. This sensation is often accompanied by anxiety and shortness of breath.

Heart palpitations are not dangerous, but they can be serious. They should only last for a few beats and should go away on their own. When someone has an episode of heart flutters, it usually lasts for 10 to 30 seconds.

If the episodes do not stop after 30 seconds or so, this could be a sign that something is very wrong. You may also experience chest pains, sweating, shortness of breath, nausea, or dizziness with heart palpitations.

Some people may feel like they are having a panic attack when experiencing these symptoms. Your pulse rate will increase when you have an episode of heart palpitations, which means your heart beats much faster than within one minute.

Causes

Doctors are not entirely sure what causes heart palpitations, though some factors increase the chance of an episode. Anyone can experience heart flutters, but they are much more common in people who have pre-existing conditions.

Health conditions such as anxiety disorders, thyroid abnormalities, high blood pressure, Cushing's disease, lung disease, and diabetes can cause heart palpitations. Other causes include caffeine intake or alcohol consumption before bedtime, which may disrupt your sleep pattern.

Also, stress hormones play a role in causing these episodes to happen. Stress can also worsen these symptoms. If you suffer from anxiety, it is important to manage your mental health well so you don't have recurrences. Certain medications can also trigger heart palpitations. For example, beta-blockers can cause tachycardia or atrial fibrillation.

Tachycardia is a condition in which the heart beats faster than usual, beating over 100 times per minute during an episode. This is considered to be a medical emergency. When you have an episode of tachycardia, your heart can stop or cause you to pass out if it does not resume its normal rhythm.

Atrial fibrillation is another common heart arrhythmia that causes episodes similar to palpitations. Other types of arrhythmias include sinus bradycardia or atrioventricular block. Palpitations are also common in people who have thyrotoxicosis, where the thyroid gland becomes hyperactive due to increased levels of thyroid hormones.

Risk Factors

The risk factors that cause heart palpitations are pretty much the same as those that increase your chance of having a heart attack or stroke. If you have high blood pressure, high cholesterol levels, diabetes, or smoke cigarettes, then you are at a greater risk of experiencing heart flutters. Other complications include stress and anxiety disorders. Heart palpitations are also common in people who have a family history of heart disease.

Symptoms of Heart Palpitations

Some of the most common symptoms associated with an episode include:

- Dizziness or lightheadedness
- Shortness of breath/feeling like you cannot breathe
- Rapid heartbeat (tachycardia) or racing heart (pounding sensation in your chest)
- Chest discomfort or tightness

Diagnosis and Treatment

There are several tests you can undergo to determine the cause of your heart palpitations. Your doctor will likely perform blood and urine tests, as well as an electrocardiogram (ECG).

An ECG involves attaching electrodes to your chest and arms with a sticky substance and using these electrodes to monitor your heartbeat and electrical activity. You may be given medicine that slows down or speeds up your heart rate so you have a better chance of experiencing symptoms of palpitations during the test. In some cases, you may receive medicines that can trigger episodes of palpitations for you to film them on video.

Your doctor will also ask about any medical conditions or family history that may increase your chances for this condition. Your doctor might prescribe medication if he or she determines that you have any underlying conditions that affect your heart rate.

Once your doctor diagnoses heart palpitations, he or she will likely recommend ways to manage the symptoms. Lifestyle changes include taking up meditation and deep breathing exercises, giving up smoking, managing stress levels, exercising regularly, eating a diet low in fats and caffeine, avoiding alcohol consumption before bedtime, etc.

You might also be prescribed medications if necessary. If you are experiencing episodes mainly at night time, ask about changing your medication dosage so it can take effect during this timeframe rather than earlier for better sleep quality.

Some lifestyle changes that may help with insomnia include planning regular sleeping hours for yourself, incorporating relaxation activities into your daily routines such as yoga or meditation, avoiding drinking caffeine after midday, and so on.

Managing Your Heart Palpitations—the Right Way

You can manage heart palpitations in several ways, but you must do it the right way for optimal effectiveness. You should also be patient when dealing with this condition because some lifestyle changes may take time to show results. Here are some helpful tips:

Stay active

Staying active is one of the best ways to manage heart palpitations. It helps lower your stress levels so you can feel less agitated and anxious. A healthy diet combined with regular exercise can help you reduce your body weight as well, which may improve the effectiveness of some medications that you are taking for this condition.

You don't have to spend long periods at the gym; start by walking more often or doing other small exercises like yoga poses during breaks at work. This way, you will slowly build momentum and become more passionate about staying fit and healthy overall.

This lifestyle choice will likely impact several aspects of your life positively in the process too, such as improving mental focus, skin appearance, etc., not just your heart condition.

Do not smoke

Smoking is detrimental to your health and may contribute to frequent episodes of heart palpitations. If you want to avoid this symptom, stay away from cigarettes, cigars, or any other tobacco products. This is one of the best ways to do it anyway because some smoking cessation medicines may cause slight fluctuations in heart rate, particularly if you already have a history of this condition.

Avoid stress triggers at all costs

Stress is another significant trigger for frequent episodes of heart palpitations. This includes stressful conversations, heated arguments, watching violent movies, or listening to angry music. You should try to relax during these scenarios by avoiding them altogether if possible and if not, taking a time-out until you feel less agitated. Then engage in slow breathing exercises while sitting down until you feel calm enough to carry on with whatever you are doing. Learn how to manage stress effectively by taking up a relaxing hobby such as painting, knitting, or playing an instrument. By all means, avoid stressful activities during work hours if at all possible because this can adversely affect your performance and also increase the chances of having a heart palpitation episode.

Apply an ice pack or cold compress

There are many reports of using ice packs and cold compresses for fast relief from symptoms related to hyperadrenergic POTS syndromes such as heart palpitations, lightheadedness, chest pain, anxiety, and shortness of breath.

To apply an ice pack or cold compress, simply put it in the freezer then remove it when needed and wrap it in a clean cloth before applying it gently on the affected areas like your neck and chest area. Do not apply ice packs directly on your skin. If you prefer, you can also use cold compresses made with chamomile tea which has calming properties that may help ease symptoms like anxiety, restlessness, and irritability.

Apply pressure to your carotid sinus area

This is one of the simplest home remedies for heart palpitations that you can try. To do this, simply lie down or sit in a comfortable position then place your index and middle finger on the sides of your neck with your fingers in line with Adam's apple and underneath the jawbone. Gently press both sides of the neck with your fingers until you feel a pulsing sensation; hold for 30 seconds then release and repeat several times per day.

Be vigilant about sleeping habits

Many people who have been diagnosed with heart palpitations reported that they usually experience their first symptoms overnight or while trying to fall asleep. You should consider going to bed early for optimal restorative sleep every night because it has been shown that those who slept less than 5 hours each night had a higher rate of developing this condition compared to those who slept for 7 hours or more nightly. If you find it hard to fall asleep at night, try turning off all lights and using a sleeping mask to help your body prepare for sleep as darkness stimulates melatonin production in the brain.

Sleep with an extra pillow

Sleeping with an extra pillow under your legs may help reduce symptoms such as heart palpitations especially if they are related to menopause or other hormonal changes. To do this, simply place a pillow or cushion under your feet while lying flat on your back in bed. Make sure you have a few pillows to choose from so that you can find the one that is most comfortable for you.

Consult a healthcare professional if symptoms worsen

If heart palpitations become chronic or last for longer intervals, make sure to talk to a medical professional about it. This way, your doctor can advise you on any treatment options that may be available such as switching medications or trying other lifestyle changes like avoiding specific substances that trigger the problem. You should also visit a physician regularly even if your heart palpitations are not severe because this will allow them to monitor you closely and see how well any therapy is working.

Managing Heart Palpitations Through Diet

Besides using medication and lifestyle changes like avoiding alcohol and caffeine, individuals who want to reduce the frequency of heart palpitations can also incorporate therapeutic foods in their diet. Here are some foods you should incorporate more into your diet:

Increase dietary fiber intake

Dietary fiber is particularly helpful for those who experience constipation as it keeps bowel movements regular and speeds up transit time through the digestive tract. This can help alleviate pressure on the intestinal walls that may contribute to heart palpitations. What's more, including soluble fibers in your diet will result in a slower release of glucose into the blood which could further reduce blood pressure levels especially if you already have high triglycerides or cholesterol. There are many simple ways to dietary fiber such as snacking on dried fruits like apricots, prunes, and figs. You can also try adding ground flaxseeds to your favorite cereal or smoothie recipe for some added fiber.

Consume magnesium-rich foods regularly

Magnesium is an essential mineral that aids in heart palpitations control by helping the heart muscle contract regularly with little to no effort required. It has been known to relax blood vessels, prevent calcium overloading in the cells, and reduce inflammation which could be another reason why it helps lessen symptoms of this condition. The only way you can get enough magnesium from foods alone is by eating lots of green leafy vegetables, whole grains, and nuts.

Consume omega-3 fatty acids for heart palpitations relief

Omega-3 fatty acids such as those found in seafood like salmon and halibut as well as some plant sources like flaxseeds, chia seeds, and walnuts can help ease the symptoms of heart palpitations by reducing inflammation levels which are linked to this condition. Omega-3s make platelets less "sticky" which will prevent them from clumping together and clotting inside blood vessels, thus preventing a stroke or heart attack. What's more, these fatty acids may also help lower blood pressure and cholesterol which can further reduce the risk of stroke or heart attack.

Eat foods that are rich in folic acid for palpitation relief

Folic acid is a type of B vitamin essential for cardiovascular health because it helps produce red blood cells which carry oxygen to the heart. It also reduces the amount of an amino acid called homocysteine found in the blood because this substance is directly linked to the narrowing of arteries thus increasing the risk of heart attack if levels are too high. Foods such as lentils, spinach, asparagus, avocado, broccoli, brussels sprouts, beans, and legumes contain a good amount of folic acid so be sure to include them in your diet at least thrice a week.

Eat foods that are rich in vitamins B and C

Fruits and vegetables like oranges, lemons, grapefruit, and strawberries contain high amounts of Vitamin C which can help ease heart palpitations by breaking down the sticky plaques found inside the arteries thus improving blood flow. Additionally, most fruits and veggies such as cucumbers, mangoes, grapefruits, strawberries, etc. also contain high levels of B Vitamins which can reduce inflammation levels and improve muscle coordination (thus reducing the number of irregular heartbeats). A good way to make sure you're getting enough vitamin B is by taking a daily multivitamin or trying snacking on foods like watermelon, broccoli, cauliflower, and sweet potatoes.

Foods to Avoid

Other types of food should be avoided to manage heart palpitations effectively. Some of these include:

Sugar and foods high in sugar

Many people do not realize how much simple sugar they consume daily until they begin keeping a food diary. Even seemingly healthy snacks such as fruit juice can contain extremely high amounts of sugar which could overload the pancreas and cause unstable blood sugar levels including those associated with diabetes or hypoglycemia. If you have been diagnosed with either of these conditions, then it is best to switch to natural sweeteners like honey or stevia rather than processed ones made from white flour and cane sugar.

Alcoholic beverages

Drinking too much alcohol can lead to high blood pressure and an irregular heartbeat which may dramatically worsen symptoms of heart palpitations. Alcohol is known to increase the production of stress hormones such as adrenaline and cortisol which can damage your heart if it becomes too abundant in your bloodstream. It also causes fluid retention, so you should limit the amount of alcohol that you consume each week to avoid serious health problems such as hypertension and obesity.

Artificial sweeteners

Saccharin, aspartame, or sucralose—all samples of artificial sweeteners—are found in many diet products today yet they could cause more harm than good especially if you already have heart palpitations.

Consumption of these substances has been linked with a greater chance of developing metabolic syndromes such as diabetes, high blood pressure, and obesity. People who are taking certain medications including antidepressants should also avoid artificial sweeteners as they may cause serious health problems.

Caffeine-rich foods or beverages

Caffeine is known to increase the heart rate which can trigger heart palpitations in some people. Aside from cola drinks, caffeine is also found in products like energy drinks and coffee. If you drink more than two cups of coffee per day, then it would be best to switch to decaf or green tea instead.

Processed meats

Processed meat like hot dogs or sausages contain preservatives that could affect the rhythm of your heartbeat once they enter your bloodstream; thus triggering unwanted palpitations. Meats like these also contain high amounts of sodium which causes bloating and fluid retention.

Foods that contain monosodium glutamate (MSG)

Monosodium glutamate is a flavor enhancer found in processed foods and meat, and it can cause adverse side effects such as headache, sweating, and heart palpitations in some people if taken in large amounts. Avoiding this substance will help you prevent the symptoms of toxicity although it is always best to consult your physician before making any significant changes to your diet just to be sure that you are doing the right thing for your condition.

We have previously discussed several nutrients that may reduce or even manage heart palpitation symptoms in natural ways, but we have not yet discussed possible foods that can make your palpitations worse. Let us now discuss some of these foods with you.

Sample Recipes

The following are some recipes that you can incorporate into your daily meals to help you manage the symptoms of heart palpitations.

Salmon and Asparagus

Ingredients:

- 2 salmon filets
- 14-oz. young potatoes
- 8 asparagus spears, trimmed and halved
- 2 handfuls cherry tomatoes
- 1 handful basil leaves
- 2 tbsp. extra-virgin olive oil
- 1 tbsp. balsamic vinegar

Instructions:

1. Heat oven to 428°F.
2. Arrange potatoes into a baking dish.
3. Drizzle potatoes with extra-virgin olive oil.
4. Roast potatoes until they have turned golden brown.
5. Place asparagus into the baking dish together with the potatoes.
6. Roast in the oven for 15 minutes.
7. Arrange cherry tomatoes and salmon among the vegetables.
8. Drizzle with balsamic vinegar and the remaining olive oil.
9. Roast until the salmon is cooked.
10. Throw in basil leaves before transferring everything to a serving dish.
11. Serve while hot.

Tahini Salmon

Instructions:

- 1/4 cup tahini
- 3 tbsp. fresh lemon juice
- 1 tsp. mashed garlic
- 1/4 tsp. salt
- 1/2 cup finely chopped cilantro
- 2 tbsp. roughly chopped toasted walnuts
- 2 tbsp. roughly chopped toasted almonds
- 1 tbsp. finely chopped onion
- 1 tsp. extra-virgin olive oil
- cayenne
- black pepper, freshly ground
- 1 lb. wild salmon skin removed, fresh or frozen

Instructions:

1. In a bowl, combine the tahini, 2 tbsp. of lemon juice, 3 tbsp. of water, mashed garlic, and 1/8 tsp. of salt; set aside
2. In a separate bowl, combine the cilantro, walnuts, almonds, onion, olive oil, cayenne, black pepper, and 1/8 tsp. of salt.
3. Fill the bottom of a steamer with water and bring it to a boil.
4. Season fish with 1 tbsp. of lemon juice.

5. Place it on a plate and put it on top of the steamer. Cover and cook, taking care to remove while the fish is still pink inside, about 3 to 4 minutes.

6. Remove the fish from the steamer, top with the tahini mixture, and then with the cilantro mixture.

7. Serve warm or at room temperature.

Seafood Stew

Ingredients:

- 2 tsp. extra-virgin olive oil
- 1 cut bulb fennel
- 2 stalks celery, chopped
- 2 cups white wine
- 1 tbsp. chopped thyme
- 1 cup chopped shallots
- 6 ounces shrimp
- 6 ounces of sea scallops
- 1/4 tsp. salt
- 1 cup chopped parsley
- 6 oz. Arctic char
- 2-1/2 cups of water

Instructions:

1. Heat a frying pan on the lowest setting. Add a small amount of oil.
2. Cook the celery, shallots, and fennel for approximately 6 minutes.
3. Pour in the wine, water, and thyme into the frying pan.
4. Wait for 10 minutes and allow it to cook.
5. Once much of the water has evaporated, add in the remaining ingredients, and wait for 2 minutes before removing it from the stove.
6. Serve and enjoy immediately.

Lemon-Baked Salmon

Ingredients:

- 2 pcs. lemons, thinly sliced
- 3 lbs. salmon filet
- kosher salt
- black pepper, freshly ground
- 6 tbsp. butter, melted, 6 tbsp.
- 2 tbsp. honey
- 3 cloves garlic, minced
- 1 tsp. thyme leaves, chopped
- 1 tsp. dried oregano
- fresh parsley, chopped, for garnish

Instructions:

1. Preheat the oven to 350°F.
2. Line a rimmed baking sheet with foil. Grease with cooking oil spray.
3. Lay lemon slices on the center of the foil.
4. Season salmon filets on both sides with kosher salt and freshly ground black pepper.
5. Place the filet on top of the lemon slices.
6. Whisk together oregano, thyme, garlic, honey, and butter in a small bowl.
7. Pour the mixture over the salmon filet.
8. Fold the foil up and around the salmon to form a packet.

9. Bake for 25 minutes or until the salmon is cooked through.
10. Switch to broil and continue cooking for 2 more minutes.
11. Garnish with chopped fresh parsley and serve hot.

Salmon with Avocados and Brussels Sprout

Ingredients:

- 2 lbs. of salmon filet, divided into 4 pieces
- 1 tsp. ground cumin
- 1 tsp. onion powder
- 1 tsp. paprika powder
- 1/2 tsp. garlic powder
- 1 tsp. chili powder
- Himalayan sea salt
- black pepper, freshly ground

Avocado sauce:

- 2 chopped avocados
- 1 lime, squeezed for the juice
- 1 tbsp. extra-virgin olive oil
- 1 tbsp. fresh minced cilantro
- 1 diced small red onion
- 1 minced garlic clove
- Himalayan sea salt to taste
- black pepper, freshly ground

Brussels sprouts:

- 3 lbs. of Brussels sprouts
- 1/2 cup raw honey
- 1/2 cup balsamic vinegar
- 1/2 cup melted coconut oil

- 1 cup dried cranberries
- Himalayan sea salt
- black pepper, freshly ground

Instructions:

To make the salmon and avocado sauce:

1. Combine cumin, onion, chili powder, garlic, and paprika seasoned with salt and pepper. Mix well before dry rubbing on the salmon.
2. Place the salmon in the fridge for 30 minutes.
3. Preheat the grill.
4. In a bowl, mash avocado until the texture becomes smooth. Pour in all the remaining ingredients and mix thoroughly.
5. Grill salmon for 5 minutes on each side or until cooked.
6. Drizzle avocado on cooked salmon.

To prepare the Brussels sprouts:

1. Preheat the oven to 375°F.
2. Mix Brussels sprouts with coconut oil. Season with salt and pepper.
3. Place vegetables on a baking sheet and roast for about 30 minutes.
4. In a separate pan, combine vinegar and honey.

5. Simmer in slow heat until it boils and thickens.
6. Drizzle them on top of the Brussels sprouts.
7. Serve with the salmon.

Asparagus with Garlic and Onions

Ingredients:

- 1/2 lb. fresh asparagus, trimmed
- 1/2 cup white onion, diced
- 3 tbsp. butter
- 1/4 cup water
- 2 cloves garlic, thinly sliced
- salt
- black pepper

Instructions:

1. Add water, asparagus, and onion into a skillet. Cover it.
2. Bring it to a boil over medium heat. Steam for about 2-5 minutes, or until the onion and asparagus are slightly tender.
3. If necessary, add a few tablespoons of water to maintain the steam.
4. After the water evaporates, add butter to the skillet.
5. Continue cooking until the asparagus and onions are lightly browned.
6. Throw in the garlic and cook for about half a minute more.
7. Add salt and pepper according to your taste.
8. Serve and enjoy while warm.

Broccoli-Kale with Avocado Toppings Rice Bowl

Ingredients:

- 1/2 avocado
- 2 cups kale
- 1 cup broccoli florets
- 1/2 cup cooked brown rice
- 1 tsp. plum vinegar
- 2 tsp. tamari
- sea salt, to taste

Instructions:

1. In a small pot, simmer broccoli florets, and kale in about 3 tbsp. of water. Cook for 2 minutes.
2. Add tamari, vinegar, and cooked brown rice. Stir to combine.
3. Transfer pot contents into a medium-sized bowl and top with sliced avocado; sprinkle a dash of sea salt to taste.
4. Serve immediately.

Stir Fry Broccoli, Onions, and Carrots

Ingredients:

- 1 tsp. light olive oil
- 1-1/2 cups onion
- 2 cups medium-sized carrots
- 6 cups medium-sized broccoli
- 2-1/2-inch broccoli florets
- 1/4 tsp. of sea salt
- 1/2 cup of water

Instructions:

1. In a pan, heat sesame oil to medium-high heat.
2. Sauté onions. Add in carrots, broccoli, florets, and then water.
3. Season with sea salt, and cover the pan to bring to a boil.
4. Lower the heat and bring to a simmer for 5 minutes.
5. Pour some soy sauce if needed.

Optional:

1. Top some pasta or rice with stir-fried vegetables.
2. Substitute other vegetables with cabbage, cauliflower, or yellow squash.
3. For additional flavor, sauté 1 tbsp. minced ginger before adding carrots.

Apple and Onion Mix

Ingredients:

- 1 medium-sized Granny Smith apple, finely diced
- 1/4 cup red onion, finely chopped
- 1/4 cup walnuts, toasted, finely chopped
- 1 tbsp. extra-virgin olive oil or walnut oil
- 1 tsp. lemon juice
- 1 tsp. honey
- 1/2 teaspoon sage, finely chopped
- a pinch of salt

Instructions:

1. Place apple dice, chopped onion, chopped walnuts, chopped sage, oil, honey, and lemon juice in a bowl.
2. Toss until all ingredients are evenly distributed and coated with honey-lemon dressing.
3. Sprinkle it with salt to taste.
4. Serve immediately.

Hearty Chicken Salad with Pasta

Ingredients:

- 8 oz. penne pasta
- 1 (6-oz.) chicken breast
- 1 cup seedless red grapes
- 1/4 cup walnut pieces
- 1 tbsp. red wine vinegar
- 1/2 cup chopped celery
- 1/2 cup Greek yogurt
- 1/2 tsp. black pepper
- 1/8 tsp. salt

Instructions:

1. Start by cooking the pasta, a small addition of cooking oil is recommended.
2. Continue cooking the pasta for 7-9 minutes before removing the water.
3. Remove the fat from the chicken and chop it into small pieces.
4. Boil some water and place the chopped chicken into it. Boil for 7 minutes.
5. Remove water from both ingredients.
6. Add both the chicken and pasta together with the rest of the ingredients.
7. Cool down before serving.

Chicken Breast Delight

Ingredients:

- 1 tsp. dried oregano
- 1/2 tsp. rosemary
- 1/2 tsp. garlic powder
- 1/8 tsp. salt
- finely ground black pepper
- 4 chicken breasts

Instructions:

1. Remove any fat from the breasts.
2. Mix the remaining ingredients in a separate container.
3. Add the mixture to either side of the chicken.
4. Prepare a frying pan, lightly oil the pan, and set the stove to medium.
5. Add the chicken to the frying pan. Cook for 3 to 5 minutes on each face.
6. Cool the chicken for a couple of minutes after cooking.
7. Serve warm.

Roast Broccoli and Salmon

Ingredients:

- 1 bunch broccoli, cut into florets
- 4 tbsp. canola oil, divided
- salt
- pepper
- 4 pcs. salmon filets, skins removed
- 1 pc. jalapeño or red Fresno chile, seeds removed, sliced into thin rings
- 2 tbsp. rice vinegar, unseasoned
- 2 tbsp. capers, drained

Instructions:

1. Preheat the oven to 400° F.
2. On a large, rimmed baking sheet, put the broccoli florets and toss in 2 tablespoons of the canola oil. Season with salt and pepper.
3. Roast the florets in the oven for 12 or 15 minutes. Toss occasionally.
4. Remove from the oven when the florets are crisp-tender and browned.
5. Gently rub the filets with 1 tablespoon of the canola oil. Season the salmon with salt and pepper.
6. Put the salmon in the middle of the baking sheet.

7. Move the florets to the sides of the baking sheet. Roast the filet for 10 to 15 minutes or until the filets turn opaque throughout.
8. In a small bowl, combine the vinegar, chile rings, and a pinch of salt.
9. Let the mixture sit for about 10 minutes so that the chile rings become somewhat softened,
10. Add the capers and the remaining tablespoon of canola oil. Add salt and pepper to taste.
11. Drizzle chile vinaigrette over the roasted broccoli and salmon just before serving.

Oat and Blueberry Pancakes with Yogurt

Ingredients:

- 2 large eggs, beaten
- 1 cup blueberries
- 1 tbsp. maple syrup
- 1/2 cup low-fat cottage cheese
- 3/4 cup plain low-fat Greek yogurt
- 1 tsp. vanilla extract
- 1 cup old-fashioned rolled oats
- cooking spray

Instructions:

1. Combine eggs, cottage cheese, vanilla, and oats in a blender and process until you obtain a smooth consistency.
2. Add the blueberries and stir them in without pulsing the blender. Divide the mixture into 6 equal portions.
3. Put a large nonstick pan over medium heat. Coat it with cooking spray.
4. Pour a portion of the batter and cook for 3 minutes. Flip it and cook the other side for another 3 minutes.
5. Get a small bowl and combine maple syrup and yogurt. Mix well. Divide the mixture into two equal parts.
6. Each pancake serving comes with a yogurt-maple syrup mixture.

Apple-and-Honeydew Smoothie

Ingredients:

- 1 pc. Gala apple, peeled and deseeded
- 4 tbsp. fresh aloe vera, peeled
- 2 cups Honeydew melon, peeled and deseeded
- 1/16 tsp. lime zest
- 1-1/2 cups ice
- 1/4 tsp. salt

Instructions:

1. Put all the ingredients in a blender.
2. Blend until smooth. Start from low to high blending. After that, stir.
3. Serve immediately.

Anti-Diabetic Smoothie

Ingredients:

- 2 cups spinach
- 2 large kale leaves
- 3/4 cup water
- 1 large frozen banana
- 1/2 cup frozen mango
- 1/2 cup frozen peach
- 1 tbsp. ground flaxseeds
- 1 tbsp. almond butter or peanut butter

Instructions:

1. Using a blender, mix the water, spinach, and kale. Increase speed until all solid particles are gone.
2. Add the rest of the ingredients. Resume blending until reaching the maximum speed.
3. Maintain the maximum speed for 30 seconds before serving.
4. Serve chilled.

Vegetable Pasta in Avocado Sauce

Ingredients:

Zucchini Pasta

- 2 zucchini
- 3 cups red and yellow cherry tomatoes
- 4 oz. pasta

Avocado Sauce

- 1/2 cup fresh parsley
- 1 tbsp. miso paste
- 1 garlic clove
- 1 avocado
- 1/4 cup olive oil
- 4 green onions
- 1/2 tsp. salt
- juice from 1 lemon
- ground pepper, to taste

Instructions:

1. To make the avocado sauce, use a blender to pulse all ingredients until smooth. Set aside.
2. In a large skillet over high heat, drizzle olive oil and cook cherry tomatoes until the skin loosens. Season with ground pepper and salt.

3. In the same skillet, add the zucchini, and avocado sauce; toss to combine.
4. To serve, season with ground pepper and salt to taste; garnish with extra tomatoes.

Conclusion

Because of how common it is, people don't usually worry about having heart palpitations. However, due to the number of possible causes of this sensation, some people feel troubled by how it feels, especially when it lasts longer than usual.

There are, however, other health conditions linked to palpitations, so it's important to get a proper diagnosis from a doctor to rule out any other possible conditions. Even a supposedly simple and common sensation such as heart palpitations could be a symptom of other health diseases.

As illustrated through this guide, one way to manage this is through proper diet and nutrition. The food items best to alleviate the symptoms of this sensation are mostly heart-healthy, so following the diet program will benefit your overall health. Just make sure that you consult first with a doctor or a nutritionist before following a diet program.

If you enjoyed this guide, please leave a review. Best of luck on your journey.

References and Helpful Links

Heart palpitations. (2017, October 18). NHS.UK. https://www.nhs.uk/conditions/heart-palpitations/.

Heart palpitations after eating: Guide to foods and conditions that cause your heart to pound. (n.d.). Flo.Health - #1 Mobile Product for Women's Health. Retrieved November 19, 2022, from https://flo.health/health-articles/diseases/heart-conditions/heart-palpitations-after-eating.

Heart palpitations: Medlineplus medical encyclopedia. (n.d.). Retrieved November 19, 2022, from https://medlineplus.gov/ency/article/003081.htm.

Heart palpitations: Symptoms, causes & treatment. (n.d.). Cleveland Clinic. Retrieved November 19, 2022, from https://my.clevelandclinic.org/health/diseases/17084-heart-palpitations.